The Battle with an Enemy Called Bipolar

The Win Over Depression

by

Rochelle D. Smith

DORRANCE
PUBLISHING CO
EST. 1920
PITTSBURGH, PENNSYLVANIA 15238

Dorrance Publishing Co
585 Alpha Drive
Suite 103
Pittsburgh, PA 15238
Visit our website at www.dorrancebookstore.com

ISBN: 978-1-6376-4395-2
eISBN: 978-1-6376-4429-4

The Story of a Great Woman
and Her Battle with Mood Disorder

Yin-Yang

Yin and Yang are two complementary principles of the Chinese philosophy: **Yin** is negative, dark, and feminine; **Yang** positive, bright, and masculine. Their interaction is referred to as "an ancient concept and symbol referring to complementary opposites"(Wikipedia).

Hence a spiritual image of a person who is affected by the disorder known as bipolar.

Introduction

This book is dedicated to a great woman who has fought a great battle. A courageous battle of the mind! This book was written for my mother, a strong and resilient woman who never allowed anything or anyone to keep her down. The challenges of my mother's life began with the loss of her mother. Following this distressing, encompassing sequence of events or rather a chain of events, there was no indication of mental challenges present. However, internally my mother was experiencing a mood disorder. This was very difficult to determine because outwardly, she always appeared very strong and unconquered by life's unrelenting displeasures.

Essentially, my mother was constantly being tormented by unresolved internal and external issues. Unfortunately, I was not able to help her resolve these mental and spiritual struggles which lied within her. Neither was I able to assist her with achieving the inner peace she so desperately desired and needed. I had to constantly remind myself that this was not a battle of her soul but a temporary affliction of the mind.

Oftentimes, I felt as if God had only supplied me with a temporary answer. A long-term solution that would end this tormenting of her mind seemed fruitless and farfetched. The tormenting of her mind had become a never-ending cycle of events. Preventing her from leading a full and normal life. Instead, she had become one filled with chaos and instability.

This book is also dedicated to those of you who have loved ones who are struggling with mental illness. Especially to those who have parents who are suffering from this adverse condition which afflicts the mind. I pray that God will give you all peace within. This book was written to highlight an illness known as bipolar. It was written to bring about healing to all who may read it. I have revealed to you one of my deepest wounds in this book.

Contents

The History of Mental Illness

According to a psychologist, mental health is defined as the ability or the absence to see oneself as others do. Moreover, it is the inability to fit or conform to what is considered the norm. Not fitting into one's environment, culture, or society where one lives. However, throughout the history of mental illness, individuals who possessed a mental illness were often misdiagnosed, mistreated, or simply overlooked.

Essentially, little has changed regarding society's perception of mental illness. Even with the advancements of therapeutic treatment and counseling within the health care system, many citizens with mental illness are not receiving the proper treatment. Despite new developments and innovative changes occurring within the mental health system, there are still many who are suffering in silence. Unfortunately, when it is time to allocate funding the mental health system lacks priority.

There is a constant awareness as well as a rise in the circulation of literature concerning mental illness shared on various social media platforms. However, we continue to ignore the needs of those who are mentally ill and intellectually challenged. All too many times they are ignored even by members of their own family. Oftentimes, left to fend for themselves. There are some who will turn to street drugs as a form of self-medicating. However, it is our misconceptions of what mental illness is comprised of as well as our cruel intentions towards those who are experiencing a mental crisis has led to them to such intolerable behaviors.

Because of this rejection which stems from members of their families these same individuals are forced to leave the safety of their own homes and roam the city streets. In search of drugs in a futile attempt to self-medicate. Failing to receive the proper mental health care in which they are so desperately in need of, the city streets become their place of refuge. However, this was one of my greatest fears. To see my mother cast out of the safety of her home. Only to roam the city streets alone and completely out of touch with reality. Finding herself subject to physical harm or unspeakable danger. Thankfully, this has never occurred. My greatest hope is that these mass killings which have occurred would shed some light on these individuals who are desperately in need of the proper medical attention. The message that I am conveying is to help provide these individuals with crisis intervention before they get to the point of wanting to harm others.

For many years, our society refused to acknowledge and/or address the problem of mental illness with medical treatment. There were a few who changed history by doing just the opposite such as Dorothy Dix, Hildegard E. Peplum, and Linda Richards, who were all nurses who stood for and brought about change within the mental health system. Simply by preventing or ending the inhumane treatment of those who were suffering from mental illness.

The research provides proof of this mistreatment of the mentally ill by providing the state with the indisputable evidence of this mistreatment then developing a structured plan that would resolve this mistreatment of the mentally ill. Truly I can attest to this mistreatment of the mentally ill as well as the misdiagnosing of these individuals. Initially, my mom had been diagnosed with anxiety and depressive disorder. Unfortunately, her disease progressed to bipolar with an affected mood disorder.

Following Hurricane Katrina she became bipolar with schizophrenic tendencies accompanied by frequent manic episodes. Often becoming delusional and experiencing periods of hallucinations with homicidal thoughts. Having the first knowledge of this dreadful disease has helped me to better cope. To better cope with this horrific disease process, it is better to equip yourself with detail knowledge and history of this illness.

Our society has and can continue to gain much knowledge by updating persistent research. It is through research that we can and will gain more insightful knowledge on just how to manage and treat mental illness. It has been through studying and performing much research that I acquired knowledge of just how progressive mental illness can become. In fact, it was there during my research that I discovered how an individual's state of mind will decline as they begin to age.

Therefore, a constant re-evaluation of the medication regimen must occur. There were many questions that would often enter my mind regarding this illness because I believed heavily in spirituality and the things of God. There is constant warfare in my mind regarding the spiritual side and the scientific occurrences.

Background

Unfortunately, my mother did not live to see her story put into production. At the ripe old age of ninety years old, my mother transitioned from this life into the next. She literally died fighting with her mental illness. Although my mother had lived to see me both rise and fall then rise again. Despite her age, the death of my mother was a hard blow to our hearts. Miss Lillie was one of the strongest and courageous women I have ever known.

Miss Lillie was one of the strongest as well as courageous women I had ever known. Enduring hardships, mental meltdowns, spiritual transitions, and heartache yet, she continued to persevere. I will never forget the day we laid her to rest. As we rolled down the streets of Slaughters, I observed as the leaves of the trees were frilling about in celebration of my mother's return to her home. Suddenly, this incredible feeling of warmth and peace took ahold of my heart. My tears begin to dry, and my spirit was up lifted and suddenly I realized that my mom was at peace and the internal battle had come to an end. The life of one of the most amazing women I had ever known had ended with peace and complete calm.

The Beginning of the Battle

When she was only sixteen years old, somehow the illness seemed to have faded away into the darkness. Like cancer, it just hid tightly away within her cells. Hiding within the very depths of her mind. Simply lying dormant waiting for the opportune time to resurface and to take complete control. I believe that this drastic transformation begins to take place in many women in the form of postpartum depression.

Especially in those mothers who are over forty years of age. Those who have previously experienced multiple births. According to the psychologist, postpartum depression follows the birth of a child. In many women, the onset of depression occurs with the conception of an unwanted child and progresses with the birth of the child. Therefore, it is important to provide a new mother with lots of emotional support. However, in Ms. Lillie's' case, the onset was during her teens and reoccurred in her forties.

Like all young children, Ms. Lillie's life began like that of any child. She was born in a two-parent household. Her mother was thirty-eight years old when she gave birth to Ms. Lillie. Her father was well into his fifties. At birth, my mother had eleven siblings and four wonderful, loving, and caring grandparents. However, at the young and tender age of eighteen months old, this all changed.

Unfortunately, my grandmother was tragically taken away in a car accident. She died of a broken neck accompanied by internal bleeding. Now, this occurred in the late 1920s. Therefore, major intervention for a broken neck was just to keep the patient stabilized. I am more than sure that the fact of her being a black woman in Slaughters, Louisiana in the 1920s reduced her odds of living from little to none. Following the death of my grandmother, a different kind of battle took place. The kind that destroys family ties.

The tiny baby girl was practically snatched from her father's arms and placed into those of her paternal grandparents. My grandfather found himself in a battle with his in-laws regarding the welfare of his eighteen-month-old daughter. The question was raised who the best provider for the child would be. My grandfather continued to battle with my grandmother's sibling over the right to keep his baby girl. However, he later forfeited his rights as a parent. He did what any father within today's society would do. He took the child to live with his parents in the countryside. Hoping that his parents would serve as a better example than himself.

My great-grandfather was a very tall, dark, proud, and superstitious man. Born in Africa a decent of the Gideon tribe. He was espoused to a very tiny Native American who was of the Cherokee tribe. She remained there in the couple's home until their deaths. Following the death of her grandparents, my mother returned to her home with her father. Once again, the battle over her welfare would return.

My great-grandparents both passed away, and once again the battle begins. This time between a loving aunt and a doting father. My mother found herself being tossed about and practically ripped from her father's grasp. During those days, it was considered inappropriate for a man to raise his daughter without a wife. Suddenly, my mother found herself amid another dilemma.

After much deliberation, Ms. Lillie ended up living with her mother's eldest sister. Now she would become a member of a new home. Unfortunately, it was there in her new home that this dreadful illness began to take hold of my mother. Consequently, it was at the ripe old age of sixteen when my mother first encounter what she called a "dream-like state." Her actual words were, "I felt as if I died." Neither one of us has come to a concise decision on what had transpired. All she can recall is walking around in a daze incapable of properly communicating with anyone.

However, there is one sure aspect of the incident that she can recollect, which is that an unknown wind blew in through the front door and something in the wind took a strong hold over her entire being. Causing her to walk around somewhat unconsciously. It was a loud scream from her cousin along with down-home prayer combined that would bring her back to reality. At that moment she would collapse into the bed and become overtaken by a force she had never encountered before.

At the age of eighteen, my mother went off to live with one of her elder siblings in Paris, California, which is located right outside of Los Angeles. While there she worked, played, and attended nursing school in Los Angeles. It was there in the heartbeat of California that my mother ran into one of her homeboys as she called him. Mr. Rhythm and Blues himself Mr. BB King.

Following him around like a schoolgirl in love. Well, that is until one night while exiting a nightclub, a 2x4 which held a flashing sign with BB's name on it fell and hit my mom in the very top of her head. Causing her to sustain a powerful blow to the center of her head. It was that blow to the head that changed the course of her life.

It was shortly after these events had occurred that my mom received a letter stating that her father was nearly at death's door. At the receipt of this letter, she decided to return home to provide consolation to her dying father. My grandfather was the decedent of a strong and prideful African from Guinea and a tiny mother who was full-blooded Cherokee. Therefore, my grandfather was not only strong but very prideful and courageous.

After just one semester in nursing school, my mother had to withdraw. Her father had become gravely ill with cancer. The old man had become confined to the bed and was losing ground. My mother tried every way to continue to revive her father but he lost the fight against cancer. Shortly after the burial of her father, my mother returned to California. This time as a short order cook in one of my uncles famous restaurants. My uncle was a wiz in business, and this venture would be no different than any of the others.

It was my mother's eldest brother who had the greatest impact on her life. He took her under his wing and molded her from a caterpillar into a beautiful butterfly. He took his responsibility as a big brother very seriously, but soon my mother's impulsiveness and anxiousness would return. It was not very long before she would end up in a place which she had long loathed, and that was

Woodville, Mississippi. She hated that place with a passion because it held nothing but gloom for her.

Woodville, Mississippi held all those dark passions that often would stir up hate and disdain for others. It was there in Woodville where my mother would fall in and out of love and decided to take on a very difficult yet different path to freedom. In addition to this, she would endure great suffering, loss, and pain. It was a place of deep, dark secrets. A place filled with death, darkness, and dread. Fortunately, her stay there would not be very long.

It was there in Woodville, Mississippi where my mother met her true love and lifelong friend, but something tragic happened to detour her path to marriage. A too familiar face showed up. It was tragedy accompanied by death. Once again, my family had experienced tragic loss. This time it would be my mother's middle sister. They were tighter than two thieves.

A matter of fact, it was because of my Aunt Bessie that my mom had decided to march all the way to the altar with this handsome, dashing man. While there at the altar, my mother received the news of her sister's untimely death. This severed her relationship and quickly brought all her notions surrounding marital bliss to an end. The dashing, well-groomed gentlemen enlisted into the military, and my mom returned to L.A. However, this would not be the end of their lifelong love affair.

Prior to my aunt's death, she and my mother had celebrated everything together. Following this, my mother had given birth to her firstborn. She was totally career driven. By this time, she had become a fabulous cook. Remember her humble beginnings were in a Waffle House owned and operated by her and her eldest brother. Who instilled a wonderful business sense into her head.

Subsequently, it would be following the tragic death and burial of my aunt that my mother would once again return to Los Angeles. This time sharing a tiny apartment with a co-worker. It was only after a few short months that that same anxiety would return, and she would leave L.A. This time her destination would be the Big Easy. This is where she became a chef and a mother.

Later that same year, my mother would enroll in cosmetology school. Now she was presented with two challenges. Number one, she was a black single female. Number two, she was now a single mother, and both were frowned upon in the 1950s. Once again, her anxiety combined with ambition would gain the best over her. It was in 1958, and once again my mother was back on the train to California. She would remain there for only five years and return to the Big Easy.

Fortunately, there in New Orleans my mother could always find work. Instantly, she became employed in the French Quarter working for a renowned Southern family. Catering and cooking was truly Ms. Lillie's forte. It was there in a tiny little restaurant she quickly began to regain her momentum. Her passion for creating French cuisine would become the vice that would keep her landing on her feet.

In 1962, she gave birth to her second child and once again with her faithful friend and teenage beau remaining at her side, but it was all very short lived. Following the birth of her middle child, Ms. Lillie reconvened her travels, and off to California she went. Leaving her past behind her to move forward to a better future.

By this time, LA was a breeding ground for anyone who was seeking out success. Ms. Lillie absolutely loved Los Angeles. It stood for everything she believed in regarding life and liberty. Let us not forget it was the perfect world for a glamorous lady like herself. In California, Ms. Lillie could live the life she always dreamed about.

Ms. Lillie's goal was to live a very successful yet peaceful existence. Finally, this goal was within her grasp. At least for a while, it seemed as if she had accomplished just that. By managing a Waffle House that was owned by her eldest brother. Cooking for others as if it were second nature to her because it was truly her first love. Amazingly, cooking was one of those exceptional gifts that she possessed from a child.

It was exactly four years later and now 1966. A very tumultuous year. The '60s had to be one of the most controversial times in American history. It was a time when great people such as Martin Luther King Jr., Malcolm X, and Muhammad Ali lived, and the Kennedy family all thrived. It was also the time of despair and loss for each one of them. In addition to this, it was the return of my mother's age-old battle with a mood disorder.

Return of the Enemy

In 1966, my mother made New Orleans, LA her home and never to returned to California again. She found stable employment and pursued her lifelong passion as a chef. I believe it was there in 1966 when the onset of depression began to set in. This time, the depression would stem from a late termed pregnancy or what doctors called postpartum depression. It was there in the year of 1966, at the age of 38, Ms. Lillie gave birth to a bouncing baby girl. That same year, she gave birth to an illness now deemed as bipolar disorder.

It would be for a sequence of years that we would move back and forward between Baton Rouge and New Orleans. It was within a time frame of twelve years. All due to this illness called bipolar disorder. In those days, the term "manic depressant" meant the death of dreams and hopes. Constant hospitalizations maybe even being institutionalized. Being institutionalized was something my mother had become all too familiar with.

In 1972, my mother became engaged to the man who is now known as my stepfather. This man endured my mother's illness like a champ. Remaining devoted not only to my mother but to her children. He withstood all the turmoil and transitioning without any complaints. As did my father. Who stood by quietly and supported us through it all.

Although it would take my mother a total of five years to totally recover from her prior setback, she did. After five years of a hiatus, Ms. Lillie left Baton Rouge, LA and returned to that old faithful city called New Orleans. Returning stronger and more determined than ever to achieve her previous goals with due diligence. At the same time, landing back on her feet and building a strong foundation for her family. Accomplishing all that she set out to do without missing a beat.

Finally, in 1976, with the birth of my niece, we returned to New Orleans to rebuild our lives within the city walls. Just for a second, life was good. For just a moment in time everything seemed perfect.

We all were off doing something that we loved because the city was filled with excitement. Ms. Lillie was off doing what she loved, and that was catering parties. I would reap the benefits every evening. Ms. Lillie would return home with all kinds of treats left over from the featured event.

In 1992, my mother returned to school and became a caregiver. For over four years she nursed and nurtured two families before retiring once again. Even after retiring, she would nurture members of the entire neighborhood. By simply preparing meals for the sick as well as those who were confined to their homes. Her giving heart would not allow her to stop sharing her gift of love and her passion for cooking.

On a final note, it was in the 1970s when my mother and my stepfather began a lifelong relationship. A relationship which lasted nearly twenty years. Like any relationship, they endured the test of time, but overall, it was a great one. One filled with friendship and walking in agreement. In the 1990s, my stepfather felt the call of death and returned to his parents' home in Houma, LA. Houma became his final resting place.

The cycle of this illness begins with my birth, and for this reason and this reason alone it left and a deep scar upon my heart. As I write this word, I must sit and pause. I literally must sit and take deep breaths as I ponder on the devastating impact this illness has had on my life. An old friend told me to stand and look back with a grateful perspective, but I find it too hard to do so. Why? Because this disease basically robbed me of the intrinsic and intimate years with my mother. Yes, time after time. My mother regained her momentum and learned to become resilient, but somehow, I still feel as if we were defeated.

My mother could single-handedly raise three amazing children as well as hold a job as a chef. Let us not forget, time and time again triumphantly arise from her manic episodes. Time and time again, I watched her recover, each time losing parts of herself. Yet she continued with her walk with God. Fellowshipping, teaching, and ministering to all who would follow and listen. The chef, the nurse, the cosmetologist, a devoted mother, grandmother, great-grandmother, and Sunday school teacher. I introduced to you an amazing woman and mother.

Chapter One
Defining the Disease Process

Let us first discuss the difference between the two diseases and the symptoms which accompany each disorder as well as their patterns. The disorder is first characterized by depression. The onset of depression can stem from many of life's disadvantages, such as loss of a job or a loved one as well as obesity. It is defined as a decrease in vital functioning. Moreover, it is further defined as a mood disturbance characterized by feelings of sadness, despair, worthlessness, and discouragement.

Depression can also be accompanied by anxiety, obsessive-compulsive disorder, as well as substance and alcohol abuse. Others are schizophrenia and eating disorders. The substance abuse can be present in many forms, such as tobacco, heroin, amphetamines, and cocaine. In addition to this, there is frequent abuse of cannabis, benzodiazepines, codeine, and cough suppressants. The misuse of prescription drugs can sometimes begin in the home. The drugs are obtained directly from your medicine cabinet.

According to psychologists, anxiety is defined as anticipation of impending danger or dread. Anxiety is further defined as a state of nervousness and restlessness as well as feelings of severe apprehension. Now, bipolar is often described as a chemical imbalance which stems from a major depressive disorder or mood disorder and a spiraling out of control into a manic state.

It has also been deemed as a mood affective disorder. One that is characterized by at least one episode of manic behavior with or without reoccurring manic episodes. Although this individual has encountered one manic episode of mania and has been diagnosed as bipolar, this same individual can be experiencing a combination of illness or symptoms that can be classified as psychotic. This means the individual is experiencing multiple disorders at one time.

For example, this individual could be diagnosed as bipolar with schizoid affective disorder or bipolar with psychotic features. In addition to this, a person can be diagnosed as bipolar with suicidal ideation or schizophrenic with suicidal ideation. Before we enter the world of psychosis and take a more in-depth look, consider mental illness.

Let us begin with learning what are some of the key triggers that lead to all mental illnesses. One of the leading triggers is emotional disturbances or emotional instability. An emotional disturbance always has been the leading contributor to any mental illness. The cycle can be triggered by the loss of a loved one. Maybe a tragic or traumatic event occurred such as loss of income or a major accident, which caused a severe physical disability.

According to the experts, an emotional disturbance is a condition exhibiting the following characteristic: inappropriate types of behavior, pervasive mood swings which incorporate sadness and depression. Others are the tendency to develop physical symptoms, eating disorders, fears, and phobias which stem from personal problems. An emotional disorder can lead to social disorders. However, the experience of long-term depression will lead to bipolar disorder, and in turn can lead to schizophrenia.

These statements are all very factual. How do I know this? Because this is the exact pattern thatledup to Ms. Lillie's development of mental illness. However, many psychiatrists defined schizoid affective disorder as a social disorder characterized as self-absorbed; the individual is restricted emotionally and is cold and indifferent. Schizophrenia is characterized as a brain disorder with this disease; a genetic predisposition can be a contributing factor as well as stress (M. Hogan, G. Smith, 2003).

These illnesses can be characterized by a mixture of delusional thoughts accompanied by frequent periods of hallucinations. Hallucinations involve hearing voices talking to or about the individual. Delusions involve believing that people on television or on the radio are speaking directly to the individual. In addition to this, the person has difficulty distinguishing between reality and fantasy. Their thinking becomes very bizarre and distorted from reality.

Furthermore, there is the loss of facial expressions, which has been deemed a flat affect. Many others will display what is termed a mask-like expression. Demonstrating or conveying a total lack of emotion. The individual may also withdraw socially from family and friends. Unfortunately, delusional behaviors can lead the individual to display very dangerous behaviors. Very high-risk behaviors that can result in negative consequences. Oftentimes ending in physical harm or even death.

According to researchers, schizophrenia involves a mixture of positive and negative features. The individual seems to lose their desire for life's pleasures. The individual loses their personal perspective and positive outlook regarding life. Most people who are affected by schizophrenia also experience personality disorder, anorexia, bulimia, and intense phobias (A. Roberts Ph.D.).

Schizophrenia is a very serious disorder. One which anticipates long-term therapy. However, this condition warrants a combination of therapies, such as antipsychotic and antidepressant medication as well as social, recreational, and occupational therapy/rehabilitation. In most cases, it will take years of therapy to properly treat and manage this illness. Why? Schizophrenia is triggered by many stressful or traumatic events. The onset occurs in the late teens or early twenties.

Schizophrenia can often become intertwined with personality disorders. These two disorders can make a very deadly combination. This form of the disorder is frequently seen in people who have been diagnosed with paranoid schizophrenia. However, there are many who exhibit borderline personality disorder. These individuals are very antisocial and display cruel intent toward those who are very close to them.

Others are very egocentric, impulsive, and obsessive. The problem persists with simple adaptation to their environment. There are two more common disorders that have been linked to schizophrenia and bipolar disorders. These are anorexia nervosa and bulimia, which are eating disorders frequently experienced by teens and many adult models. However, there have been a few recent cases of adults who are experiencing eating disorders.

One of the most popular recorded cases of bulimia was that of Princess Diana, who persistently struggled with issues with her physical appearance. The desire to be perceived as tall, beautiful, and thin can become an extreme obsession that later turns into illness. The evidence of these disorders can prove the beginning onset of schizophrenia or bipolar disorder. Even in an adult's onset, either of these deadly disorders can be present. They are sometimes reoccurring during manic episodes. The individual either chooses not to eat or simply forgets because of the extreme case of mania.

Many teens will alter their eating habits by substituting or trading healthy habits for unusual eating patterns. Whereas anorexia entails incorporating poor to usual eating habits such as substituting high-calorie food for healthy choices. The individual may consume crackers and ketchup as opposed to eating bread. Other extreme habits are eating starch out of the box or even graham crackers blended with yogurt.

In contrast to anorexia, most people affected by bulimia find ways to frequently purge following the consumption of an extremely large meal. These individuals are frequent binge eaters. However, following the binge, they will cause themselves to vomit. In addition to this, the individual will frequently instill rectal enemas.

Finally, we will discuss phobias and obsessive-compulsive disorders which often accompany schizophrenia. Through years of experience obtained from working within the mental health division, very few of them have acquired this disease via genetic disposition. The average person affected by a mental disorder has acquired it through some type of traumatic experience, extreme stress, or years of drug abuse. However, what all these tragic events seem to have in common is the onset of psychosis.

In contrast, or rather on the spiritual side, I once heard a preacher describe bipolar as demonic possession. One personality is defined as the individual and their inborn and innate desire to function like a normal human being. The other personality has been characterized as some form of demon that has possessed the person totally, which is demonstrated with loud outbursts, disheveled appearance, and unorganized thought pattern. The use of foul language, lashing out at loved ones, and the inability to practice proper hygiene.

Many ancient civilizations believed that the only solution to freeing a tormented soul of an evil spirit was to drill a hole into the skull. This would allow the being to escape and at the same time release this individual's mind and soul from the constant tormenting of their spirit. I am more than sure that few patients would survive this type of surgical intervention. Yet the villagers thought that this was an effective method of cleansing their village of unwanted evil spirits.

At this point in my life, I do not know what to believe. I have come to realize that there is mostly a change in mood and character that takes place during the manic episode. In contrast to the outspoken, tongue-lashing individual there is another side. On one side there is this kind, gentle and giving person. A very God-fearing woman and the other is a defiant, very oppositional individual.

The person who is experiencing the manic symptoms can often turn into an individual who becomes physically combative, argumentative, and very confrontational, as well as someone who persistently demonstrates a total lack of fear. These diseases do not discriminate. These diseases can affect people of all races, creed, and color as well as affect people of various social economic backgrounds and financial status. In addition, there is an absence of bias regarding educational background and status.

Chapter Two

Ms. Lillie

Ms. Lillie was born in the year 1928. In a little town in Louisiana called Slaughters which was near the Louisiana/Mississippi state line. Her life began like that of any other normal child. Ms. Lillie grew up in a two-parent home with the support of maternal and paternal grandparents. She was the youngest of twelve children. Her mother Mary was a cook and a gospel singer, and her father Wilson was a hard-working field hand. By the time my mother was born, many of her siblings had become young adults.

One day while riding in the car with her uncle as well as her mother and two of her elder sisters, an accident occurred. She was told that one of her uncles was driving the car. Apparently, he fell asleep behind the wheel and the car veered off the road. Prior to this, my grandmother turned around and handed my mother to her eldest sister. At the time of the accident, my mother was only eighteen months old. My grandmother was the only one injured in the accident. However, she was transported to the hospital where she later died of a broken neck. Ms. Lillie would reside with her father until she was five or six years old.

Unfortunately, a dispute regarding her well-being sparked, and off she went to her paternal grandparents' home. Now, their little home was in the small town of Woodville, Mississippi. In Woodville, my mother would be surrounded by nearly all her family. Everyone thought that this would be a great move. It was there in her grandparents' home where healing would take place.

My great-grandparents possessed the ability to nurture those old wounds. I do not know exactly what took place in their home. I would like to believe that the healing power of my great African ancestors was brought forward through my great-grandfather. Maybe it was the spirituality of the Cherokee nation, which my great-grandmother possessed. I do not have an inkling of an idea. All I know is whatever the chosen method, it worked!

Unfortunately, her stay would be short because her grandparents were well stricken in age. Her parental grandmother was a Native American woman who suffered from a severe case of diabetes. Now, her grandfather was one hundred percent African and very superstitious. He was not going to allow a child to remain in his home without a woman present. So, my mother went back home to her father.

Consequently, another dispute surfaced regarding the care of my mother. This time she went off to live with her aunt, which was her mother's sister. My grandfather became very furious about this. It would be there in my great aunt's home that this illness would take hold of my mother. She was the ripe old age of sixteen when the onset of this dreadful disease occurred. Not knowing just what had overtaken her.

Apparently, my mother began to wander about in a trance tracking the very footsteps of one of her elder cousins. At the sight of my mother's condition, she screamed and attracted the attention of everyone in the house. By this time the screams had caught her aunt's attention who was at that time busy in the kitchen cooking. At the sound of the scream, my great aunt fell upon her knees and began to pray. My mother then turned around and fell onto the bed where she would remain for days. There she remained upon her bed of affliction until she would finally awaken from her trance.

Chapter Three
The Entry of the Enemy

I cannot tell you the exact date or time in which the enemy entered our lives; I just know it did. The enemy stole our joy, peace, and happiness. It would practically destroy our home and family. This same enemy tried to rob us of our mother. The enemy divided our family and left us vulnerable and frail. Prior to this, this same enemy arriving, my family was happy and united. My mother was always a proud, well-dressed, and hard-working woman. My mother was so well groomed that she refused to allow one hair upon her head to be out of place. She was always perfectly groomed in the latest fashion.

A doting mother, who loved to spend quality time with her children, our home would be so clean you could practically eat off the floors. I always felt as if God had a special purpose for my family because we seemed to endure things that no other family was enduring. I presume my outlook was adopted from my mother's perception of her life. There is an old saying which states, "When you are a child, your perception and view of life is acquired through your mother's eyes."

This wisdom that she instilled in you is obtained via her life experiences. Therefore, if her view of life is somehow altered or distorted due to mental illness, this will somehow affect the child's view of life. My mother would always say, "Whatever affects the mother will affect the child." Do not get me

9

wrong, this does not always apply to mental illness. I do not agree with the statement that bipolar is an inherited trait. My mother did not inherit this dreadful disorder. This illness was caused by a sequence of traumatic events.

First being separation anxiety and post-traumatic disorder due to the sudden death of her mother. The second was depression due to a family tragedy. The third was due to physical exhaustion from working three jobs to support her family. Therefore, I do not agree with what the experts suggest. Why? Because time and time again my mother was misdiagnosed and never properly treated—of course, her lack of proper insurance had nothing to do with this. I know that a lot of sociologists and psychiatrists will disagree with my analogy, but this is what I believe.

Most of my knowledge regarding mental illness was solely gained through experience. Over fifty years of enduring my mother's illness just standing by powerlessly watching it unfold layer by layer. To all of you who believe that you are at risk for this horrible illness, search out your families' history. You may not be at risk for future episodes of mental illness. After many years of research, I have learned that the beginning of any mental illness stems from depression.

Depression can lead to a vicious cycle of uncontrolled episodes of mania with several attempts of suicide. I recall a movie starring Diana Ross, who portrayed the role of a medical student. While attending medical school, she was stricken with schizophrenia and became catatonic. Prior to this catatonic state, she became pregnant. Yet, she maintained zero memory of the conception and birth of her daughter. The character remained in a catatonic state for over twenty years. She was totally unaware of her daughter's existence and because of this the little girl refused to acknowledge her mother.

Furthermore, the little girl refused to acknowledge that she possessed the same qualities and characteristics resembling those of her mother. She had never encountered the presence of that highly remarkable ingenious of the medical student. She was only made aware of the mother who was catatonic and who later struggled with her medication regiment.

This dreadful illness which this young woman had acquired became so overwhelming that it would somehow subdue her youth. Unfortunately, leaving her mother in a state of suspended animation was the only thing that the little girl could identify with. Instead, the child only imagines she possessed was those of a mother who was so broken in spirit that she commenced to a catatonic state. A state of mind which left her as a shell of a person. A mother who could not express any form of motherly love? I would often compare myself to this fictional character. However, they are some exceptions. Like the fact that my mom overcompensated by smothering her children with love and affection. Her number one goal was to keep us safe from all harm and danger.

Often I would experience those same feelings of betrayal and discontentment. All brought about by a disease neither of us could control. Unlike the little girl in the movie, my mother once could demonstrate love as well as receiving it. This is an example of how this illness can diminish a child's pride, dignity, and self-esteem. All you are left with is a series of identity crises and ongoing internal struggles. Oftentimes, a child who is raised by a parent who encounters and suffers from mental illness endures lots of ridicule. You are labeled as different instead of unique, simply because others are ignorant of the effects of this horrible illness and its lasting effects. We are never really accepted by our peers and loved ones. The price is high, and the cost is infinite.

Consequently, at a very young age, you learn to become a fighter, self-reliant with the use of the defense mechanism to get through difficult situations. As a matter of fact, you spend lots of time trying to forget those past episodes of your life which are filled with pain. No longer considering or entertaining those hurtful or painful thoughts blocking out reality. On the contrary, you simmer on more joyful and happy thoughts. As time began to progress, you began to seek out a new family, by establishing new friendships and acquaintances.

However, she would consistently take on several different personas and demonstrated such behaviors as becoming very rebellious, ungrateful, unthankful, and outspoken. Many times, trying to identify with the popular crowd and identifying with others experiencing pain. Oftentimes turning to individuals who were seeking out drugs and alcohol to self-medicate to block out past experiences as well as God as a form of pain relievers.

On the other hand, I hated parts of my life and always was trying to change it. Struggling with myself and my beliefs, becoming an overachiever. This brought about the use of the defense mechanism and very risky behavior. As a teenager, I became very rebellious and took lots of dangerous risks in my life.

Because of the shame and embarrassment, we became very private and isolated avoiding conversation that involved my mother.

Everyone was too busy to notice that I was out of control. We thought that no one understood this illness including members of our family. As a matter of fact, if it had not been for the grace of God, I do not know what we would have become of us. I now know that our lives were guided by the hand of God. Truly, his grace and mercy overshadowed our lives.

What society called abnormal had become normal for my family because no one was reaching out to rescue us from the damages that this illness had brought into our lives. Each one of us began to seek out and search for a family other than our own family that would accept us with all our flaws. My mother had been hospitalized time and time again, and not one psychiatrist or therapist was wise enough to provide our family with group therapy. The Bible states, "in all you're getting get knowledge and understanding with this wisdom."

Chapter Four
Vow of Silence

The fact that my mother was bipolar with schizophrenic tendencies was devastating to us. We did not share this information with anyone. No one could get that close to us. Therefore, we became more self-reliant and independent; an example of this is: When I was six years old, my mom escorted me to the dentist office and told me to call home upon completion of my examination.

However, upon completion of the examination, I leaped out of the chair and walked to the counter, opened my coin purse, and paid the receptionist. Everyone in the dentist office was astonished by this. Then I walked from the dentist office to our tiny apartment. My mother was amazed by this. She always seemed to cling to us as though; we kept her sane.

Unfortunately, my mother never allowed herself to really have a social life. She worked from sunup to sundown. I now know that this played a large role in the progression of her disease process. She worked and functioned as a cook in the French Quarter always overworked and underpaid. The money never seemed enough to meet the bills. There was always more month than money. We were unaware of just how bad things were. That was until my mom would get ill then we would begin to understand.

Prior to her breakdown, she would appear so good at managing our finances but, it seemed as if things were quite the opposite. There would be times of mismanagement and misappropriation of funds. This would occur during her times of mania. My mom was so busy struggling to make a perfect life for us. We hardly noticed any difference until she had become dreadfully ill.

Unfortunately, my mother received very little support from our local community. Instead, she was often mocked and ridiculed. Many members of our community walked in total ignorance regarding mental illness and the major impact that it had imposed on my family or anyone else's family for that fact. Instead of embracing who she was and what she stood for as a human being as well as offering some form of assistance to our family.

Maybe someone could have extended a helping hand by attempting to guide her in the direction of shelter and/or mental help services of which she was so desperately in need. They were ashamed of my mom and refused to associate with us. We were treated as an outcast among them. We were struggling and in need of help. Only one of my mother's nephews along with his godmother would reach out and provide a lending hand.

Fortunately, there was a small remnant in the form of my mother's sibling that would reach out and give us a hand. My mom was and remained a very prideful person. She would always clothe herself and children in the fine apparel never wanting or asking for help. The only help she would barely accept was from her siblings in Baton Rouge, LA. They loved us dearly and always would come and rescue us from the claws of the enemy.

Fortunately, my family was very religious, and growing up in a religious atmosphere can sometimes be very difficult. It has its ups and downs. There are somethings that are not discussed among the members of an African-American home, the household, and mental illness is concerned as a family tragedy. It was years before I could finally understand exactly just what being bipolar entailed. The only time we would discuss my mom's illness was when my aunts and uncles wanted to interrogate us concerning my mother's illness.

Instantly, we knew when this occurred exactly what time it was. We would recognize by the signs and symptoms of mania that it was time for her to be readmitted to the hospital. This would always be a very horrific experience for my siblings and me because this process of admittance to the hospital brought us a lot of grief and anxiety. Why, you ask? Well, my aunt would acquire a mental health warrant and then contact the police. In turn, the police department would show up and apply handcuffs to my wrist then escort my mother to the mental institution via a police car.

However, this was very humiliating for us. Instantly, my mother would become hostile and began speaking very loudly. Finally, she would become combative with the officers, and a physical struggle would take place. We would have to stand by and watch this horrific scene unfold with all our friends and neighbors standing by watching. This was not the way a person suffering from mental illness should have been subdued.

We lived within a very close-knit community. So, of course, everyone would come out to observe her departure. We were so young and endured criticism from our peers as well as family members as if we had caused this illness. My so-called friends would laugh and mock me. Certain members of our family would laugh and call my mom crazy. Of course, I would be fighting mad! No one ever considered how we felt or what type of impact this would have on us. Not even my mother. I do not blame her for these traumatic experiences, because she could not control her manic episodes.

Upon recovery, all memories pertaining to her manic episode were a loss. The thoughts of inner spiritual war have always lingering in the back of my mind. Yet, I still wonder within myself, what does it mean to be bipolar? Is it like someone having a split personality or is it the devil tormenting the mind of your loved one? I am aware that there are personality changes. There is the humble, sweet person, and then there is this out of control, full of rage person.

Chapter Five

Internal Suffering

It has been approximately one year following the impact of Katrina's devastation, and my mom has been hospitalized exactly seven times within a two-year span. These were unlike the hospitalization of the past. These were a direct result of Katrina's aftermath.

Now, my mom has suffered from mental illness since I was about the age of three or four. I can remember sitting on my father's knee at my aunt's kitchen table listening attentively to their discussion of my mom's illness. I cannot tell you what caused her first manic exposed. But I can reveal to you several of the traumatic events which may have contributed to this horrible illness and it is taking a chokehold on my family.

Unfortunately, leaving my poor defenseless mother feeling totally out of sorts. When my mother was about eighteen months old, she was in a motor vehicle accident that claimed the life of me and mother. Her father fought to keep her at home but lost that battle to my great-grandparents. Mostly my great-grandfather, who was a great big and tall African filled with African pride. Now, my grandpa, Wilson, was no easy win. He was known as a fearless man and one who terrorized the town as well as the blacks in his community. My great-grandmother was a very tiny Native American lady who was quite outspoken. There is no doubt in my mind who initiated this custody battle. After several years of being tossed about, my aunt, Amanda, who was my grandmother's eldest sister, came forward and stated that my grandmother made her promise to raise my mother.

Apparently, my grandmother lived for several minutes after being transported to the hospital and this promise was made upon her deathbed. My grandfather did not believe it but allowed them to take her after giving them hell! This was the second tragedy that occurred following the death of my grandmother. My grandfather was several years older than my grandmother. Therefore, as Jacob loved Joseph and did not want to part with him, my grandfather did not want to be separated from his eighteen-month-old daughter. He believed in keeping his family together. My aunts were all young women and, like my grandfather, disagreed with this decision. I believe my grandfather hated them for breaking up his family. I was told that the death of my grandmother brought about drastic changes to all their lives.

My mother never adjusted to this change of environment as well as, this sudden separation from her parents. There is without any reasonable doubt evidence of separation anxiety. Oh, let us get back to the story. It was there in my great aunts' home where my mother's first episode of mania occurred. One day, when she was sixteen years old, my mother was babysitting one of her cousins, and while passing the doorway she felt a very hot breeze enter the house.

Suddenly, my mother began to pace about behind one of her elder cousins. My mom said, "I had this bad feeling come over me as if I had died." Well, her cousin screamed out for her mother, and immediately she bowed down and began to pray. My mother turned around and walked to the bed and collapsed. It was several days later before she would recover. Experts would say that this was the beginning of the onset of what is now called schizophrenia. It was the last they had seen of this occurrence.

Until several years later, when my mom recovered, she wrote a letter to her older brother who resided in Paris, California. He sent her a train ticket, and her adventure began. While in California, she came across an old friend and he invited her to one of his concerts. This was none other than Mr. B.B. King. While exiting the concert alongside Mr. King, an iron rod fell from across the doorway and struck her on top of her head. I believe this had a definite impact on the return of her illness.

Two years later, my grandfather was sentenced to prison for stabbing a guy to death. While in prison he was diagnosed with some type of cancer. He was given a pardon based on a letter my mom wrote to Governor Huey P. Long. She had just moved to California and was attending nursing school while living with my brother and his wife. Once pardoned, my grandfather sent for her and she returned to Slaughter, LA. There she would take care of my grandfather until he died. So, at the age of eighteen, my mom found herself absent from both parents. Because of his death, she became very close to her sister and moved to Mississippi.

However, it may have been about nine years later when the death of her favorite sister occurred. Her life was stolen from her by mad man. My mom went back to California and then back to Louisiana. Three children and several jobs later, my mom became ill again. We had no idea what happened! All we knew was that our mom was sick again and we had no control over this illness.

Once and again, she was returning to Jackson State Institution and would remain there for several months. We would visit her every weekend. She would chain smoke Salem100s and shake uncontrollably. It would be several months before we would have her in our lives again. Still, no one ever considered how this would affect me as well as my siblings.

Jackson State Mental Institution was one of the worst facilities I had ever encountered. Visiting this institution was one of the most horrific experiences of my life. It was like viewing a scene from a 1930s' movie about an insane asylum. People were pacing about talking to themselves and doing all types of undesirable things. My aunt and uncle tried their best to give us a normal life and meaningful existence while my mom was away, but inside each one of us was crushed.

Deep down inside it felt as if my insides were screaming out for help. You see, I was always the one who would cling to my mother. My sister and I would cry at the very presence of our mother's emotional state and her physical appearance. She would come out walking like a zombie, very heavily sedated. It would be difficult to communicate with her, but I guess this would be better than hearing her yelling out obscenities to the voices in her head as well as her pacing about and fighting the air. I guess therefore she would come home and flush the pills down the toilet.

Chapter Six

A Change in Environment

After the third hospitalization, my uncle finally decided to purchase a home for us in Baton Rouge. We stayed there only for a short time. My mother quickly decided to return to the Big Easy. This return brought on changes that we all would never forget. My family remained there until I was about nine or ten years of age. Once settling into a new place, my mom would work herself into another nervous breakdown. This time my uncles convinced her to admit herself. She was not very happy with these arrangements, but there were no alternative measures. So again, our lives would be turned upside down.

It would not be so bad. My aunt and uncle would take turns providing for us. Well, until my uncle died suddenly due to a hunting accident. This too had a tragic effect on my family. We all were devastated by his death. My mother had lost her number one supporter and we had loss and uncles and a mentor. They would keep us involved in church activities and garden duties. You see, both my uncle and auntie owned very large farmers with gardens. So, we were very well provided for.

The transition of moving from city to country life brought about big changes for us. Living within a small town in Louisiana was much different than living in a big city. A smaller community would provide us with a solid foundation. It is the place where we found God and he found us. My uncle was a big deacon in the church, and my auntie was a very well-established missionary. My entire family attended a small Baptist church. Every one of us had to attend each Sunday service. We would be there all day long on Sunday. Let us not forget Bible study on Tuesday, prayer on Thursday. Saturdays was set aside strictly for missionary duties as well as hayrides on the back of my uncle's old Ford pickup.

After several months my mom would recover. She would leave my aunt's house to go out and re-establish her own place and began her healing process. I have always admired her for her strength and resilience. My mother had the ability to make a tremendous come back. She would regain her strength and composure, obtain her children, and return to work. We wore the best of clothes and rarely went without food.

When she would become ill, she would forget to pay her bills and have us walk the streets both day and night searching for a new place to live. By some miracle from God, we would never be homeless nor harmed. We would go and live with her godmother from time to time until she could reestablish herself. Later, my family would return to New Orleans, and a miracle occurred. Immediately, my mom would return to work and a normal routine.

Chapter Seven

Sustaining

We were introduced to a great man of God. Pastor Benson McGee was a great man of God who taught us great lessons concerning the physical and spiritual side of life. From him, we obtained insightful knowledge concerning the word of God. It was there at the House of Faith Church of God in Christ where my mother would receive her healing. It was through the word of God and the laying on of hands that my mother would maintain her sanity. There she would function as a pastor's aide and a mother of the Church as well as a Sunday school teacher.

Only once while attending this place would she relapse. For over fifteen years my mother remained manic free. Not until Hurricane Katrina had arrived and blessed us with her furious presents would my mother's illness returns with a vengeance. We had enjoyed fifteen years of total sanity, absolute zero regression. It was there at the convention center following those long dark nights and during that weeklong escapade would her illness return. She was not alone, because there were many more collapsing under the pressure which we had to endure following the storm of the century. Now, you are the judge! Is it an enemy of the mind or vexation of the soul?

Since Katrina, my mother has been hospitalized thirteen times within a ten-year span. Following admittance to four different hospitalizations and eleven manic episodes and three different physicians later, yet my mother remained unstable. Those continuous unpredictable occurrences and changes in my mother's behavior, as well as paranoid and suspicious episodes, seemed to return with a vengeance.

Prior to Katrina, my mother basically maintained her own home and social life with occasional help from her children. She had held several positions as a caretaker for the elderly. Now my mother had been functioning, living, loving and as an independent with minimal assistance from others. Following her last hospitalization, her speech became slurred and very rapid. This was a direct side effect of psychotropic medication therapy.

Nevertheless, my mother remained unable to focus or concentrate for long periods of time. Her thought process was rapid with rapid speech patterns and loose association. Her clothes would be uncoordinated and very colorful. Also, she would wander about mindlessly both day and night. There was the absence of total self-control. She would get angry in an instant with ever-present hallucinations and delusions with combativeness.

Finally, after eleven hospitalizations, four psychiatrists, and frequent changes of medication, my mother was considered stable. Now, she could hold formal conversations without the racing of her thoughts and speech. Yet there was the constant presence of upper body tremors. She could perform her daily living activities and attend an adult day program. We tried to place her in a group home with others who had similar disorders; through prayer, there was a great improvement, but she not totally healed.

Only for a short time was she able to hold one thought at a time without her thoughts racing about. Her speech had become less rapid and slurred. Yet her mind and soul remained somewhat tormented. Throughout my stay here in Texas, I have sought out help for my mother, yet the results were the same. The private industry is interested in private dollars and the public industry is interested in federal dollars.

No one seems to care or at least offer small increments of compassion. It is always business as usual. Not one doctor bothered to contact her primary physician or to obtain a psychiatric history. Everyone continued to remind us of the HIPPA laws. Never acknowledging our concerns, but simply disregarding our thoughts and interests. Only one hospital included the family as part of my mother's therapy. The others did what they had considered as right for our mother. She was handed off from group home to group home without proper acknowledgment of her family. We love our mother and only wanted what was best for her.

Chapter Eight
Under Control

Following the fifteen manic episodes due to lack of proper treatment, I resulted to having a crisis team to do follow-up treatment by making home visits; this included the nurse and physician. Also, she would attend an outpatient program. The stress had finally caught up with me in the form of a tumor. Therefore, I could no longer follow through with my mom's care. She was left in the hands of the system. This was the greatest mistake my family and I had made. Adult protection got involved, and we were all treated as if we were criminals.

Later, through prayer, rest, and restoration, I regained my strength and recovered from the effects of medication and the tumor. I sought out an attorney and obtained "power of attorney"; with this I could regain control of my mother's care. To all who are providing care for a loved one, do not give up! You must continue to fast and pray, always seeking and pursuing godly knowledge and divine intervention. Also, seek out a good attorney. Work together as a family; do not leave it up to one family member to carry the load. It will take each one of you to accomplish this task.

Consequently, this illness will place a great strain on your family. So, again I say to you, pray much and seek out the help of a professional organization that can provide you with a great deal of assistance. Most of all, do not leave your loved ones alone; do not leave their future in the hands of cold and careless people. They are considered as just a number, not a person or classified by their psychiatric condition.

Throughout my life's' experiences I have found that there is a very thin line between the battle of the mind and the battle of the spirit. What affects your mind will most definitely affect one's spirit. There is no separation between the two. The mind and body and soul are all joined together. I say this because the mind and spirit are one.

It is impossible to separate the one from another. I have always heard the repeated phrase that "the eyes are the window to the soul." Only death will separate the soul from the body. Believe it or not, this statement consists of overwhelming truth, because through the eyes the mind perceives and interrupts what is considered true; if the mind is disturbed or its ability to perceive is somehow altered then your visual perception is distorted.

Unfortunately, there are so many unethical people lurking about seeking to deceive the disabled and mentally ill. If you can provide home care for your family members, please do so. This will save you a lifetime of heartache and grief; if you must find a facility for your loved one, please takes your time and thoroughly research the facility as well as investigate.

Chapter Nine
A Daughter's Perspective

My mother had to perform time and time again. Now, she was doing so with less emotional support than ever before. I was very uneasy about this.

When I was a child, I was often ridiculed, mocked, and teased to scorn because of my mother's illness. This would frequently occur in my neighborhood, church, and school. My so-called friends would spread rumors of my illness throughout the classroom setting, leaving me with feelings of alienation and humility. I refused to allow this to hamper my relationship with others continuing with my normal childhood endeavors and associations.

Oftentimes, I would find myself being divided between two worlds—the city life which I loved then the country life which I loathed at the time—because of the absence of my mother's presence. I cannot begin to describe to you the pain which I had endured as a direct result of my mother's illness. The pain of standing by and observing your mother's state of mind suddenly declined from normal to abnormal. To stand by and watch our lives begin to spiral out of control. To observe the person who protects you and keeps you safe become unable to do so.

Standing by helplessly and watching her lose total control of her mind, but at the same time sustaining her children. We would be idly standing by while she would be warring with the voices in her head in any futile attempt to obtain sustainability. We would often endure the loss of income and had to start all over again from the beginning. The admittance to the psychiatric fa-cility was always a horrific experience for all of us. There would be a temporary loss of our sole provider. The absence of my mother's strong presence, smile and laughter were awful, but somehow, we would make it through. I would like to believe it was through perseverance, fasting, and praying because we did not receive any therapy or counseling to helps us heal or recover from my mother's illness.

The endurance of constant changes in our environment with frequent periods of introduction to new relationships had begun to take a toll on us. We had to return to old familiar places, such as my uncle and aunt's home. It had become a haven for us. A unique and stable environment frequently visited because we would spend our summers with them. If it had not been for my mother's sibling I don't know where we would end up. There was an absence of fear, only the presence of sadness and tears. I became aware of exactly what mental illness was very early on in life. Not just what mental illness was, but what the definition of a mental institution was and what it constitutes.

Nevertheless a trip to Jackson State Hospital remained one of my worst life experiences. It left a negative imprint on my memory. The visitation room was massive. The place would be filled with sick people pacing about the room. Many holding conversations with invisible people as they would pace about the large room filled with cigarette smoke. Others sitting in si-lence with noticeable fine tremors or shaking uncontrollably because of the side effect of the antipsychotic medications they were taking. My mother would be walking toward us while holding a cigarette in her grasp with her hands shaking uncontrollably.

Oftentimes, I would wonder just how my mom was sustained and able to regain the normal usage of her mind. Well, the spiritual side of me says that it was the help of the good Lord. I would like to think that it was through the intervention of prayer and fasting, not mere modern-day medication because my mother would always throw her medications in the trash. She hated the way her body would respond to the medication because it would always slow her down. My mother was a cook by trade. While working in the kitchen, she needed to move very quickly, and the medication would not allow her to do so. Therefore, it would always end up in the trash.

I tell you the truth; I have endured so much hardness. There were many times when I thought that I would not be able to survive another one of my mother's manic episodes. After enduring year after year of all too numerous of her episodes, I had grown to hate this disease, and at the very mentioning of it, I would cringe. Now, even at the age of forty-seven I cringe when my mom began to exert any sign or symptoms of mania. No matter how hard I worked at trying to overcome my fear of this disease, at the slight appearance of any symptom, my fears would return.

After many years of tolling with the idea, I have finally concluded that my mother truly has no control over her illness or its disease process. I have debated with myself and others regarding this illness for years. It has literally taken many years of maturing and studying to fully understand this disease. Fortunately, I have crossed the path of many wisemen whom have helped me work through my doubts as well as overcome my fears. Aiding me in dealing with my own internal struggle and debate over what was valid and what was not. Finally, I had to let go of the struggle and give in to modern medicine.

Surrendering my mother over to strangers was never an easy task. No, it was quite difficult to do. Living in a new place among unfamiliar people and practices can sometimes take lots of time to adjust. This was an emotionally draining task. However, it was not until the 1990s that my family would be open to and receive holistic therapy. It was long after I had become a nurse and was more knowledgeable about this disease and its effects on the family; that I would even consider anything outside of traditional psychiatric help. There were times when I would resent my mother. I thought that she should stand strong and resist this awful disease. I was wrong. Repeatedly, I would ask her "Don't you feel when you are getting sick?" If I could see the physical symptoms surely she should be able to recognize the symptoms.

Unfortunately, this never occurred. My mother never recognized the symptoms. You ask, have I questioned God? I say to you a million times, why? Why did it have to be my mother? Why was my family chosen to endure such a tragic illness, and will my mother ever totally recover from it? Repeatedly, I have asked God why and how, yet he has failed to answer me. Have I become exhausted with the process of enduring the mental health system? Yes! Have I been discouraged, disillusioned, and totally fed up with this illness? Yes! I have always desired a normal mother who led a normal life just like everyone else. I hated this illness with a passion. It represented something worse than death to me. It represents something dark and painful. However, God somehow desires a different plan for my life and that of my mother.

Time and time again, I have asked God why he allowed this dreadful disease to befall my mother. Why did he choose my family to endure something as disruptive as a mental illness to afflict my mother and subdue my family? Why didn't he heal her right away? Why did he forsake us? Our lives were supposed to be as normal as that of any other child growing up in the city.

Chapter Ten
Return of the Manic Episodes

Mania is characterized as a mood disorder. A mood disorder is exemplified as a sequence of unstable gestures and emotions. Mostly, it is a state of extreme emotional excitement as well as hyperactivity accompanied by frequent periods of agitation. Oftentimes, mania can stem from episodes of severe depression. This type of behavior can sometimes become very explosive, and the only therapeutic method to resolve it is medication therapy.

Many psychiatrists will result in giving their patients a cocktail which consists of 1 milligram of Halper (Haldol), 1 milligram of Ativan (lorazepam), and 1 milligram of Benadryl. This combination of medication will correct any type of psychotic episodes. Recently, I discovered that an individual with one or more manic episodes without the accompaniment of depression is deemed depressive, but an individual with one or more mood escalations are deemed bipolar.

During my many years of researching these disorders—these are all interesting findings—I have found that many of these individuals who suffer from severe mental illness have adapted the art of manipulation. Manipulative behaviors are found in many individuals who have experienced long-term mental illness. The manipulative behavior is their way of gaining a sense of control over others. It is one adaptive pattern or rather a way to make up for the loss of control over their lives.

Fortunately, there was one unique characteristic that my mother would demonstrate prior to a manic episode. She would always pick green leaves off the trees and collect them as well as China balls and place them in the sink to soak. This was always our indication that a manic episode was soon to come. When asked, "Mom, why are you doing this?" She would simply reply, "I am blocking attacks from the enemy." Her favorite word was, "I am closing doors, and someone is fighting against me."

Unfortunately, I had to endure my mother's manic attacks and episodes too often to Keep track. However, it was those last episodes that were the worst of them all. Once she hopped into an 18-wheeler with a man and went to Kroger's then called me demanding that I come and pick her up. During a separate incident, she hopped into a car with a stranger and entered the store and commenced shopping. Following this, she stood in the line with her basket demanding that someone other than herself pay the bill!

Once again, I had to have my mother admitted to the hospital, but this time, I would be met with resistance. Finally, I met with the staff at the facility and was told that my mother needed constant monitoring, medical supervision, and stabilization of her care. During her brief stays within this facility, the doctor formulates what he thought was a bright idea. What he suggested, was to completely take my mother off her medication regimen, to place her on a new regimen because of his actions she became nearly catatonic. Following this foul up, I retained power of attorney and had my mother placed into a long-term nursing facility. By this time, I had become totally distraught by this action of the mental health system.

After, placement in the long-term facility what I discovered next was shocking. What I thought was a quality living facility was instead a very dreadful place. While there, my mother experienced another manic episode, and she was dropped off at one of the county facilities alone. To my surprise, I was awakened by a telephone call from my mother. She had been sitting in the emergency room in Ben Taube hospital all night long without an attendant to accompany her. No one bothered to call and make me aware of her status. Well, I got dressed and sped over to the hospital. I was furious!

Once arriving, I was informed by one of the nurses that they were relocating my mother. She was going to be moved another facility which was located adjacent to the hospital. While walking across the breezeway to another facility, my mother began to unleash her anger and frustration out on me; because of this the receptionist refused to allow me to sign my mother into the facility. Fortunately, there was a psychiatrist standing nearby who overheard my mother ranting and raving and immediately had her admitted to the facility.

Prior to admission, my mother got into a physical altercation with a younger patient. I mean literally. I got a glance of hands swinging back and forth than suddenly from the corner of my eye, I could see fists flying behind the glass window. Totally unaware that it was my mother engaged in a dispute with another patient. I tell you the truth! My mother had become a person who I was very unfamiliar with. One weekend while visiting a family member she began to shout out the window "why wait for him to slit their throats. I could slit their throats myself." Once again, my mom returned to the hospital.

It had now been eight years following hurricane Katrina, and my mom was eighty-five years old. Her condition had become worse. Well, let's just say we have learned to live with this condition. Ms. Lillie has now been a tenant of the nursing home for over three years now. She calls constantly, making formal request to be removed from the nursing home. My heart aches at every request, but I know that I cannot manage her care. It takes a team of trained individuals working together to manage mental illness. The nursing home experience has been exhausting, yet a blessing in disguise.

Initially, my family refuted any suggestions that were geared toward nursing home placement, but now we have come to terms with our final decision. Prior to placement, no one in my home could obtain a restful night of sleep. We had to stay awake and listen very attentively to my mother's every move; if not she would have slipped right out the door without a trace. This had occurred upon two separate occasions.

Once she disappeared into my subdivision. We had to search the entire day and a large part of the evening for her. My son took to the streets riding his bicycle. Lo and behold, he found her sitting in a young couple's garage totally out of sorts. Her final disappearing act included a ride back to our home in a police car. The officer was not only very informed but immediately recognized the signs and symptoms of mental illness. While, helping to achieve calmness he told me that his father-in-law had experienced this same illness. I was so thankful that the officer possessed insightful knowledge regarding this awful illness.

Instead, of brushing us off or causing a fiasco he help and not hinder the process. The officer was very kind, considerate as well as very knowledgeable regarding mood disorder. This was something that I had not experience in the past. He made a quick analysis then recommended that I have my mother committed. At that time, I was not ready to accept the truth that my mother would never return to her former self. Her illness along with her strong will and sense of independence had become very challenging to manage.

Chapter Eleven
Institutionalized

In August of 2014, I had to relocate my mom. Unfortunately, a patient became manic during the night and physically beat his roommate to death. Somehow, my mother became aware of this and became fixated on death. Now, she had demonstrated symptoms of paranoid schizophrenia as well as pressured speech, loose association, and flight of ideas which all were classic signs of mania. Always in a state of constant fear and panic for her life. The panic attacks stem from apprehension regarding a potentially life-threatening scenario.

According to the experts, the panic attack involved disorganization of her personality, which caused an increase in motor activity. A decrease in the ability to rest and relax as well as distorted perceptions concerning reality. My mother became unable to communicate and even function appropriately. Once again, I had to have my mom committed to a mental health facility. However, this facility would differ from all the rest. Number one, the unit manager would not allow me to have my mom committed. She had to volunteer for commitment.

Secondly, they did not force their patients to take their medication. Nor did they offer any type of medical intervention such as an intramuscular injection to prevent mania. No, they just simply allow the patients to walk around totally out of their minds. Once a court order is obtained then they would use very subtle attempts for medication compliance. Previous, hospitalization allowed me to be accustomed to my mother receiving immediate medical intervention upon arrival. Yes, she was never allowed to walk around completely out of her mind. Why? It is the medication which gradually assists the patient to return to reality.

In turn, it allows them to fully participate in therapeutic sessions which aids the patient in recovery. I was told not to send my mother back to her former place of residency. So, after ten days of therapy and several failed attempts at finding a great place for my mother to live, the caseworker found a real hellish place for my mother to live. I knew from the very beginning that this was a very bad move.

After residing there for only six weeks, my mother would have an altercation with a very large twenty-two-year-old night nurse who felt the need to slap and trip my mom to the floor. Not only did she physically and mentally abuse my mother, but she later called the police. This young woman proceeded to keep me on the telephone for a total of four hours. Now, mind you, I called emergency services and they refused to remove my mother from the facility. The police officer stated. "That my mother was upset but not manic or irate." Therefore, the nurse had to embellish the story that she had previously told me.

Later that morning, I received a telephone call from the staff informing me that my mother was being transferred to a facility clear out of Houston. These words infuriate me. After only six weeks there my mother would be returning to another psychiatric unit. I agreed only because my mother needed to be transferred to a more conducive environment. One that would cater' to her specific illness. Following this, I was informed by the director of nursing that my mother would not be returning to their facility. It seemed as if the young woman's words seemed to supersede those of an elderly patient. The reason was that my mother suffered from a mental illness.

One of the most important lessons that I learned during this hospitalization was how psychological factors can contribute to as well as have a fatal impact on one's health. My mother was experiencing multiple anxiety attacks, which led to an increase in heart rate and change in the rhythm. While hospitalized in Midland, Texas, my mother acquired a heart condition, atrial fibrillation to be exact, and was placed on Xarelto to help regulate her heart rate.

Xarelto is an antiarrhythmic drug as well as a blood thinner. This condition resulted from a constant increase in anxiety, which was accompanied by a series of panic attacks which in turn caused an increase in her heart rate(Anxiety is one of the leading causes of heart attacks).

Subsequently, anxiety can lead to dehydration, insomnia, and weight loss as well as a mental confusion and a lack of judgment and denial of realistic danger, which had become my mother's passion. Oftentimes, anxiety and panic attacks can sometimes go hand and hand, and my mother was suffering from both. Furthermore, anxiety can lead to changes in her behavior such as aggression, excessive spending, hyperactivity, and grandiose acts. Each of these described the behavior that my mother had been demonstrating for years.

Afterward, she was transferred from the geriatric unit to ICU where she would remain for several days then later was transferred to another unit. I received absolutely no help from the case workers there regarding placement for my mom. It took me exactly two weeks to find my mother another long-term facility to reside in. We ended up securing a room in the same place where this had all begun. A rehabilitation/long-term care facility. The place that initially recommended that we place my mother in a home. It was there in the rehabilitation facility where my mother's health began to decline. She had experienced several falls and one single hemorrhage that would reduce her down to a shell of a person.

Prior to this placement, my mom was allowed to have a 72-hour therapeutic home visit. We would often travel back and forth to Louisiana. Providing her with some form of sanity and stability. It was an attempt to snap her back into reality by re-orientating her to familiar surroundings. When we could no longer take her out on the therapeutic leave, I would take her out on the weekend just to come over for a solid home-cooked meal.

Chapter Twelve
Evidence of Physical Changes

It is now the 10th year anniversary following Hurricane Katrina. The event that transformed my mother from bipolar to schizoaffective mood disorder as well as an accelerated case of dementia. By this time, Ms. Lillie is approaching eighty-seven, and her health is beginning to decline. Following many years of her body enduring the effects of psychotropic drugs, the sides effects of the medication was beginning o take its toll on her body.

Ms. Lillie's gait had become very unsteady, and because of this she had endured several falls. Encountering the falls led to several head injuries which led to Parkinson's and cerebral palsy which resulted in tremors of the hand and feet with persistent drooling. In addition to this, she became wheelchair-bound having to relearn how to walk with a walker. Not only this, both the combination of the psychotropic drugs along with anticoagulant meds brought about several TIAs (transit ischemic attacks).

Anticoagulants seem to have cause just as many side effects as the psychotropic drugs. The first bad drug experience was with the combination of Depakote and Zestril psychotropic drugs. After many years of working with clients, I thought that Cogentin was the wonder drug for counteracting the negative side effects of these drugs, but Cogentin seem not to have any impact against these drugs.

The second bad drug experience was with Xarelto, which led to the TIAs and persistent bleeding and coumadin which caused her to encounter seizures. One afternoon, My mother went to the dentist office to have a simple denture repair and ended up with a surgical extraction which led to a hemorrhage. Thirdly, there occurred a persistent cough, which is a side effect of Lisinopril, a blood pressure medication. Finally, there was Lipitor.

This drug serves as an anticholesteremic drug. medication. The adverse effects of Lipitor differed from that of the others but were just as detrimental to her health as were the others. Lipitor brought about such physical changes as loss of hair, upset stomach, loss of appetite, and progressive joint degeneration. Now, do not get me wrong, for someone who may be healthy this drug may not induce or rather produce the same adverse effects. On the other hand, if you are someone currently experiencing a state of decline, this is not the drug for you.

Following several months of this so-called therapeutic regimen, my mother became somewhat of an invalid. No longer walking independently. Instead, she once again became wheelchair-bound. Not able to mustard up enough strength to push the chair or even properly in steer the chair in the right direction. The physician told me that my mother had declined significantly and that she was on a persistent downward spiral. This was a very difficult thing to have to stand by and watch the utter decline of my mother. Therefore, I stepped in and began to make changes.

First, I made a few inquiries and evoked hospice to come in and take over her care. Therefore, I would have another set of eyes and ears to look out for my mother. In addition to this, the facilities nursing staff was no longer considered as the sole providers of her care. The second move was to discontinue her current medication regimen, which happened to a work like a charm. After several weeks of being off several of those so-called life-sustaining drugs, my mother encountered an astounding recovery. Well, not 100%, but she was functioning at her maximum capacity, and I was very thankful.

The culprit was never a physical enemy, but on the contrary, an enemy which lived within her mind. Something dark and diabolical seemed to live with her. Often triggering negative thoughts, which in turn would trigger negative actions.

Something way deep inside her mind simply refused to allow her to live a normal life. Those same triggers seemed to show up more often than usual. Blocking positive thoughts and allowing her to share only a few good years of total sanity with her loved ones.

Over the years, I would sit by and watch as this process repeated itself. It would gradually enter in beginning with acceleration then slowly declining and tapering off. This dreadful process would take place suddenly then fade away into the darkness. In the same manner it would enter, it would dissipate. Leaving everyone shaken and bewildered. Each time it entered; it would take away a part of my loving mother.

Although my mother had endured many setbacks and faced many challenges, somehow this disorder never seemed to have shattered her faith or belief in God. It was never allowed to hold her down neither did it prevent her from moving forward. Throughout the years, she remained a devout and devoted Christian. Each time she would recover, she would appear to be stronger than ever before.

Chapter Thirteen

Triggers

A trigger. It is helpful to first identify those stressors which trigger your depression. Avoiding these triggers will serve as a mechanism that will later prevent manic episodes. One of the major issues with bipolar disorder is mood disorientation. This is how the new title or rather name for bipolar disorder was formed. Hence, mood destabilization or rather mood disorder. With this the person's mood escalation ranges from euphoria and escalates to a form of major to manic depression.

Consequently, mania will result from some type of trigger which serves as an internal or external stimulus which activates the "flight or fright theory." During manic episodes, the individuals will experience an increase in heart rate, blood pressure, pulse, and breathing as well as muscle rigidity or rather muscle tensing. Recognizing the extreme responses that result in dramatic or volatile emotions can produce a state of stability with the absence of further intervention.

Recently, I have found that a degree of uninterrupted boredom can also serve as a trigger that will and can alter an individual's state of sanctity. However, the mental impact is based on the degree and frequency of the boredom. Once you have identified the triggers that impact your mood, you will need to find constructive ways to deal with your emotions which express themselves in the form of anger, sadness, joy, grief, and fear. Oftentimes, people find sanctuary in creative arts such as music, painting, or dancing. One of my mother's all-time favorites was arts and crafts. She often would find serenity in knitting and making jewelry.

Chapter Fourteen
Coping with Mental Illness

Let us begin by first identifying the signs and symptoms of stress. According to the psychologist, the following may vary among individuals. Sign and symptoms may begin with a lack of appetite, attention deficit (in the ability to concentrate), or short attention span. Others are insomnia(in the ability to sleep), period of high anxiety, followed by frequent chest pain accompanied by panic attacks, extreme sadness, which leads to depression or impending feeling of loss of self-control. Furthermore, there are periods of irritability and frequent visitation of mood swings accompanied by migraines.

Once again, these all are classic and realistic signs and symptoms of stress which will all lead to depression and mood disorder. Therefore, it is pertinent that you seek out treatment to help you to face and deal with responsibilities, problems, or difficulties, in a realistic, successful, and calm manner: However, coping with mental illness is never an easy task. On the contrary, it is quite the opposite.

Sydney Younger man-Cole, RN suggests the following: that one of the major goals which you establish should be toward coping with mental illness. Not only this, but that the individual who is suffering from this illness should participate in a structured plan which is geared toward the prevention or reduction of stress as well restoration of the normal chemical processes of the brain. However, like everything else, these so-called coping methods are sub-divided into positive and negative coping skills.

Most importantly, instituting a set of positive coping skills will contribute to a quick recovery from future crisis. Positive coping skills are listed as the following:

Chapter Fifteen

Stress

Stress is your body's emotional and physical response and reaction to stimuli. In other words, it is your body's response to the present demands of your world. Stressors are events or conditions in your surroundings that may trigger stress. However, stressors present themselves in two forms or rather two classifications of stress: acute and chronic stress. To give you a more detail explanation: One major stressor which was the contributing factors to my mother's illness and relapses was overworking. The other was ignoring and avoiding hurtful feelings. A major one was a denial of her illness, which hindered her potential to achieve optimal and therapeutic success.

Recently, the Mayo Clinic revealed to us a more detailed explanation of the two classifications of stress. According to the experts, "your body response to stressors depends on whether the stressor is new which classified as acute stress or whether the stressor has been around for a longer time which is classified as chronic stress"(https://www.mayoclinic.org/).

Managing stress can sometimes become a very difficult task. An identifying stressor is a key to achieving a successful recovery as well as controlling these same stressors. Whether it is dismantling a difficult partnership or dissolving a long-term relationship. Identifying stressors is a potential road toward total recovery. For many individuals, the workplace serves as the number one stressor in their lives and others in their immediate environment serve as both a stressor and a trigger. Many identifiable stressors are in the home. Others are found in a church environment. Believe it or not, many pastors and church officials can validate this information.

Coping strategies refer to the specific efforts, both behavioral and psychological, that people employ to master, tolerate, reduce, or minimize stressful events. Experts suggest problem-focused coping that target the causes of stress in practical ways which tackle the problem or stressful situation that is causing stress, consequently directly reducing the stress. Problem-focused strategies aim to remove or reduce the cause of the stressor.

Subsequently, acquiring coping skills is one of the preferred strategies for reducing the impact of a stressor. Coping skills are methods a person can use to deal with stressful situations. Obtaining and maintaining good coping skills does take practice. However, utilizing these skills becomes easier over time. Most importantly, good coping skills make for good mental health wellness. Some good coping skills: Learn to balance your daily activities and therefore balance your life.

Chapter Sixteen
Anxiety

Let us take a more in-depth look into anxiety and the deep-seated issues that may trigger our anxiety. Our society has frequently defined anxiety as abnormal behavior. However, there are many very licensed professionals who would gladly provide you with a more refreshing outlook on anxiety. Simply by providing us with a more descriptive point of view on what is classified as a quote-unquote normal behavior or abnormal anxiety. Why? Because the average American at one point or another will experience some form of a traumatic event. One that will trigger some form of anxiety.

Although the documentary also pointed out the importance of recognizing when anxiety transitions into an overt or overpowering behavior. Where an individual loses complete control over their actions/behavior and no longer holds a grasp on reality. One that will produce all the symptoms of what incorporates a panic attack or two. What are the symptoms of anxiety? Persistent and uncontrolled nervousness increases heart rate and respiration, perfuse sweating, and racing thoughts.

There is a video that everyone who is affected by these should review. It is a unique video that goes into detail about both disorders. It will provide you with an amazingly in-depth look into the world of anxiety disorder and panic attacks. One which provides a wide range of points of view. Not only this, but the documentary provided us with the baseline data which determines when the symptoms have progressed from experiencing a normal panic attack to the occurrence of a more progressive or rather chronic disorder. A disorder that could transition into something more debilitating and psychologically paralyzing. Simply by leaving a person hiding in the shadows. Moreover, confined or imprisoned within the walls of their very own home.

The documentary focused on all aspects of these conditions such as biology, physiological, and environmental factors. All three factors can and will have a direct impact on a person's ability to remain focused on reality. The endocrine system alone holds the key to physical factors that contributes to our ability to maintaining a stable existence. The statistical data provided by the documentary is staggering. To learn that over 32 million people are affected or at least encounter some form of anxiety, as well as eight out of ten people experiencing some form of a panic attack, was mind-blowing. However, the stats are very consistent with the present behaviors which several members of our society exhibit.

Dr. Shulman and Dr. Goldstein had some very interesting views on how to approach and treat phobias. There are many who would dispute their analogy regarding facing your fears head-on. However, I agree with the suggestion to first identify the deep-seated causes which trigger the behavior then pursue a solution. The subsequent therapy to treat the phobia by facing the fear head-on is a very risky technique to use. One might suggest that this sort of treatment could induce a traumatic stress disorder. Therefore, instead of curing the patient you will find yourself faced with a secondary illness more challenging than the original diagnosis.

The subsequent goal should be to carefully plan out treatment along with a therapeutic regime that would be geared toward a cure. One that will return the individual to some form of normalcy. Do I believe in medication as a form of therapy? Yes, I do. Therapy alone is not always the solution for everyone affected by these dreadful disorders. There are many who will not benefit from therapeutic measures along but a combination of holistic therapy.

Fortunately, due to innovations in science and modern medicine, we as members of a thriving society no longer must suffer in silence. There are therapeutic solutions to this age-old problem. Therefore, it is of the utmost importance that you seek out help for yourself or your family member who is suffering from a chronic anxiety disorder. Please do not allow them to suffer through this alone.

Chapter Seventeen
Panic Attacks

First, let me begin by reminding you that anxiety is a normal response to a stressor. However, if you are experiencing frequent, persistent anxiety attacks, this is not considered a normal occurrence. It seems as if panic attacks, and chronic anxiety go hand and hand. Yes, frequent anxiety attacks can eventually trigger a panic attack.

Those reoccurring feelings of complete loss of control accompanied by uncontrollable racing thoughts and possibly feelings of impending death. Each of these symptoms can be a normal occurrence if you are truly experiencing a life-threatening evident. Even if you are reliving some form of a traumatic life-changing event such as the occurrence of a natural disaster in the form of a hurricane, tornado, forest fire or even an earthquake, it could all trigger thoughts and feelings previously experienced that are buried deep inside yourself. Let me assure you of this one thing: What you are experiencing is not an uncommon or unnatural response.

On the contrary, these are all very natural psychological, biological, and physiological responses to an environmental trigger; this environmental trigger has posed a potential safety threat to your immediate surrounding. Leaving you with feelings of apprehension and disillusion. However, prolonged, or frequently visited panic attacks warrant immediate medical attention.

Consequently, the endurance of persistent panic attacks can lead to crucial physically and psychologically debilitating symptoms. Leading to frequent periods of isolation along with bouts of paranoia that can result in self-con-finement and or imprisonment in one's own home.

Many prominent psychologists feel that the goal to successfully overcom-ing your fears is to face your fears head-on. I do not advise this as a method of treatment for anyone who suffers from phobias. However, I do suggest that you first seek out the help of a professional therapist. Facing this form of illness alone is not the answer to achieving an optimal quality of life.

Chapter Eighteen
Avoiding Stressors

Physical activity is one of the leading methods of reducing stress. A daily physical regimen will help to not only reduce but control the amount of stress you allow to enter your mind. In addition to exercising, begin your day with yoga as well as an hour of meditation. Rise up early in the morning and get started before other members of your household rise. This will help eliminate the previous day's stressors and therefore not allow you to begin a new day filled with anxiety. Moreover, it allows you to spend quiet time with yourself.

One sure-fire method for achieving tranquility and restoring peace of mind is spending quiet alone. Quiet time will allow you to gain a better perspective on the previous day's events and help you to come up with more creative ways to avoid those same stressors. Seek out an environment that is conducive to restoring your energy. While there, allocate a few moments toward meditating.

Meditation is another technique that will help to alleviate stress. In addition to this, meditation will help you to start the day off fresh and anew. Another great intervention is acquiring adequate sleep and rest. Try to avoid staying up too late watching television. Prepare yourself for rest by exercising or meditating prior to ending your day. A good night's rest can help you to wake feeling fresh and totally rejuvenated.

Other essential tools for achieving optimum mental health are acquiring a hobby. My mother found solace in hobbies such as sewing, jewelry making, knitting, and spirituality. Out of all these, her walk with God took precedent and allowed her to regain sanity. She was also a big advocate for reading. My mother would spend hours reading books. One of her all-time favorite lists of novels were written by Harlequin. She must have read every Harlequin novel ever written and sold.

Chapter Nineteen
Taking Action

Taking action does not mean eliminating everyone and everything in your life. What it means is gaining control over those issues or people you interact with who contribute to the negative energy in your life. It is essential that you limit if not exclude the amount of time you spend with these individuals. This is accomplished by simply limiting or excluding the amount of time you expose yourself to the stressor. Or that idea that negative idea or relationship that you continue to ponder upon. The longer you ponder or continue with the relationship, consequently, the longer you will allow the negativity to remain and contribute to your life and lifestyle, and the longer your life will continue to spiral out of control. This person or persons are not worth your sanity. You know exactly the kind of people I am suggesting to you. The ones who manipulate and coerce you into performing negative tasks or promote negative activity which triggers a setback. I do not care if they are a lover or a friend. Even if they are a longtime friend or family member. Get them out of your lives.

What I am saying here is stop opening yourself up to those people, places, and things which lead you into a crisis. Many times, a crisis can stem from rejection or low self-esteem which comes from receiving criticism from people whom we love and esteem. So, do not allow others to destroy your self-esteem. I would rather that you seek out new friends than remain with old ones who destroy your self-esteem.

Therefore, at all costs avoid those loved ones or so-called friends or even church members who eat away at your self-esteem. Those who defame or devalue you. Give them a gift. The gift of goodbye. Avoid those intense and unstable environments as well as those volatile and intense emotions which lead to the situation you cannot control.

The goal here is to do everything that contributes and builds your esteem. To take control of your life and your health. However, this means constantly taking self-inventory. It may also mean taking measures or steps to change your value system or your ethics and morals. Taking on a new path as well as a new direction.

Change the people you interact with and the places you used to go. Leaving you with no other choice but to seek out new friends and new places. Seeking those people and places that are conducive to your quality of life. However, if you are unhappy, change those things which make you unable. Is it something physical like hair or body contour eating away at you? Well, body contour can be changed through diet and exercise.

Maintaining a healthy diet can alter how you feel inside and begin to show on the outside. Exercise can alter not just the body but the mind. Providing you with feelings of goodness inside and out. Watching what you consume via dietary consumption can play a major role in your overall mental and physical health. The goal here is to achieve optimal health status as well as a sense of accomplishing something good for yourself. Aiding you in walking away with a sense of worthiness and improved self-esteem.

First, you must believe in yourself that you can achieve any and everything that you put your mind to achieving. Plant your feet into position and stand tall and firm in your convictions. Promote yourself and all that you believe in. Do not allow yourself to become bored or tired of your new regiment. It is essential to gradually implement changes into your routine that will help you to maintain your newfound status. Go to the internet and download healthy cookbooks.

Go and search out new and creative recipes. Eat out at whole food or vegan restaurants. Instead of constantly consuming fast or bad foods. Snack healthy. Look up new exercise routines on the internet or go to the gym and speak with a trainer to gain insightful ideas. Do not allow yourself to fall into a slump.

Chapter Twenty
Achieving Change

Achieving change is never easy. It comes along with time and strategic planning. It does not take a great mind to do so. All it takes is a made-up mind to help you achieve your therapeutic goal. Yes, it can be very challenging, and no, it does not occur overnight. Oftentimes, it takes a team to determine individuals who have outlined a plan that has been devised solely for yourself.

Constructing a plan or devising long-term and short-term goals can be accomplished in several ways utilizing a few methods. This can be accomplished by you, your spouse, or your children, but the best way to accomplish this is through your psychiatrist or psychologist. Moreover, even your caseworker, pastor, or therapeutic team members can help achieve this task. Make sure your plan is a modest one. Ensure your goals are realistic and achievable and not forfeited. All goals should be measurable and obtainable.

To achieve the change, you must first be willing to commit yourself to the process. Secondly, you must develop a plan on how you will pursue change. However, changing your environment is never easy. When you grow accustomed to a certain type of surrounding or community and interacting with a certain group of people, this can present you with a challenge. Just brace yourself and know that change is needed to achieve normalcy.

Hopefully by this time you have surrounded yourself with a group or a team of well-rounded individuals who are willing and capable of helping you to achieve success. A failed attempt often results in a setback. However, a setback is not the end of the world. Just consider it as a learning experience and avoid future futile attempts that will lead you in a backward or downward direction. The steps are simple. Just take out the time to alter your lifestyle. Love yourself enough to do so quickly.

Chapter Twenty-One
Setting Boundaries

Boundaries are based on principles, values, and rules which we all live by. However, when it comes right down to implementing or setting boundaries, we all seem to fall short. Let us take it a step further. When it comes to your personal space, it is important to set boundaries or rather limits or draws a fine line between yourself and people who practice unhealthy lifestyles. However, setting boundaries should become a life skill that is practiced daily.

In the beginning, it may seem like a very unpleasant task, but after sitting down and evaluating the pros and the cons, you will find this task to be less complex than you had previously thought. Setting boundaries or limits is not rocket science. Every individual is entitled to their personal space as well as enforcing limitation on others regarding that personal space. Setting boundaries is a way of separating yourself from individuals who are demanding, controlling, as well as criticizing, pushy, abusive, intrusive, and judgmental.

Just think, sit back, and weigh the outcomes. Would you rather be confined to a psychiatric unit or in the comfort of your own home? Remember there is a fine line between sanity and insanity. Therefore, setting boundaries should be incorporated into your list of long-term goals. Setting boundaries is a form of protecting yourself from individuals who contribute to the periods of mood destabilization and who take advantage of your otherwise fragile state of mind. However, many of us have set boundaries or limitations on such individuals, yet somehow along the way these boundaries were dismantled or torn completed down.

We all have a need to, according to Pastor, Paul D. Landrew. You may have to repair those boundaries or reconstruct those broken boundaries in order that you may live a life free of destabilization, chaos, and disorder. To quote Pastor Landrew, "Do not let your guard down in order to compromise." Keep your guard up and your boundaries in place.

Pastor Landrew suggests, "Many of us build up a tolerance for certain behaviors" that we should otherwise interject; if it bothers you, put an end to it. Immediately! Your suffering from a mental illness does not give anyone the right to take advantage of you. On the contrary, this is one of the main rationales for putting boundaries into place.

How are boundaries depleted or torn down? Number one, by putting others before ourselves. Secondly, by giving into negative desires. Thirdly, by being pressured into the belief that we are jeopardizing our relationship with loved ones or friends by not compromising or giving into their ideas. The experts have classified boundaries as the following: physical, mental, material, sexual, emotional, and spiritual as well as financial boundaries. Do not lend what you do not have. On a different note, if there is someone forcing their sexual preferences on you and you are not willing to perform this sexual act, dissolve the relationship immediately.

Chapter Twenty-Two
Healing

First and foremost, achieving change is a part of the holistic healing process. When it comes to healing, there are so many aspects as well as various current viewpoints regarding the subject. There are many view healing from a religious standpoint. Others view healing as something that can be achieved through the law of self-preservation. It can also be achieved through medicinal or psychological therapies.

In contrast to this, healing is often perceived as a form of art or expression achieved through touch and verbal expression. However, each of these definitions are correct. Why? Because healing is an art that can be expressed through touch and speech. In addition to this, healing can be achieved through the law of self-preservation. It can also be established and maintained with modern medicine and years of psychological therapy. Nevertheless, at some point in time, there must be a balance achieved between each of these.

It takes a certain measure of faith and self-preservation to achieve healing within oneself. Meaning, you must be just a little selfish for healing to take place. It takes a certain amount of time set aside for yourself to become totally healed. This sometimes means withdrawing yourself from others as well as changing your daily or even weekly routine with others. Simply speaking, you must set aside time for yourself. Changing your perspective regarding yourself as well as your current belief systems. Oftentimes, it will mean changing your overall perception regarding life and how you perceive life.

Let us begin to take an in-depth look into the power of healing oneself. Beginning with changing our outlook regarding healing and self-preservation. The first step to achieving healing is to begin by focusing on yourself. First, your mindset.

Secondly, your present physical state. Your entire regimen must be focused on self. Once you have achieved this then you can focus on how your state of being will affect those who love you the most.

Throughout time, healing was achieved via some form of touch or verbal communication. Today, healing is achieved through the art of touch, which is deemed as Energy Therapy. Through touch, the negative energy is removed from your body and discarded or transformed into positive energy, and therefore healing is achieved. This is achieved through a mind, body, and spirit because you first must believe to achieve healing.

In Asia, Reiki, as it is called, is a technique performed daily. The art of touch and meditation combined has been proven to promote optimal health. Daily meditation aids in soothing the mind. The art of touch convinces the mind that the body has been healed. However, the art of therapeutic touch is one of the most visible examples of an increased acceptance of psychic healing in health care.

What does this have to do with me? You must first believe that healing is obtainable. Second, you must initiate the steps toward achieving healing. Whatever method you may choose, at some point, there must be a balance between your mind, body, and spirit.

The art of spiritual healing is accomplished through a balance of mind, body, and spirit. In order for you may achieve a balance between your health and wellbeing. You must nurture the whole being. You or your loved one cannot and will not achieve success without first doing so. The goal is to gain both harmony and balance within the body.

The first demonstration or rather form of healing was noted in the scriptures. Healing is considered an ancient art. It can be sorted out and found within every country as well as upon every continent, but do you believe? Are you willing to believe that healing is achievable simply byfirst believing that healing is obtainable and by changing what and how you feel about the subject? Right now, at this very second, there is someone staggering about mindless simply because they do not believe. Now, let us discuss faith and the belief of faith healing.

In Christianity, it is believed that healing is a proven technique achieved by the laying on of hands. In addition to this, it is also believed that healing can be achieved and maintained through a regimen of daily prayer and meditation. According to Bible scholars, God heals people through the power of the Holy Spirit; faith healing often involves the laying on of hands. It is also called supernatural healing, divine healing, and miracle healing which all flows from God. Therefore, "healing is a gift of love that flows directly from the heart of our Father in Heaven. It is God's will to heal" (1 John 4:16).

Subsequently, it does not matter what method you choose. The goal here is to choose. Choose some type of method that will help you to regain yourself. Remember the process of choosing a method is the first step to recognizing and acknowledging that there is a problem that needs a solution. Therefore, my advice to you is to choose wisely. Whatever the method you choose. Whether it is touch, faith, therapy, or medication or maybe a combination of methods. Please choose wisely, because you are truly the only one who will have to live with the outcome of your choice.

Consequently, my family chose medicinal, spiritual, and therapeutic methods as our choices. In the long run, our choice was the smartest. Although my mother later in life encountered a few major setbacks which were due to circumstances beyond our control, we still chose rightly and now our mother has returned to her normal state of relevant functionality. Yes, she is still under the care of a psychologist as well as currently maintaining a strict medication regiment, but she is maintaining and independently functional.

Chapter Twenty-Three

Restoration

What is restoration and how do we achieve it? According to Cambridge, restoration is the returning of something or someone to their original state. "Through the redeeming work of Jesus Christ, both humanity and creation are capable of being restored." The action that we will be focusing on is returning yourself or a loved one to their former self or to a better site of mind. The goal and plan are to restore you within a better place, or condition. This will entail repairing, fixing, or mending you or your loved one to a state of reconditioning or rehabilitation.

Subsequently, this will entail the rebuilding and reconstruction of your views and perceptions. Simply speaking, performing an overhaul. Through the utilization of therapeutic methods which may or may not consist of the redevelopment of your mind. This applies to all the individuals who are impacted by mental illness and the challenges that accompany this illness or are present upon course of this disease process. However, we will refer to this as a therapeutic renovation or a psychological overhaul.

Chapter Twenty-Four
Living with Mental Illness

Living with mental illness is no longer the death sentence it once was. When we think about the past, those images of patients pacing about the insane asylum seem to come to mind. Others are thoughts of patients who are permanently institutionalized sitting alone and suffering in silence. Well, those days are long gone, and this is no longer the case. Presently, there are now wonderful, well-structured facilities within the private sector that are awesome at restoring one's mental health.

What many of these facilities are offering is the opportunity to experience outstanding and award-winning services. Administered by a team of unique individuals who are experienced in providing healthy and therapeutic interventions that will help restore your faith in the mental health system. Unfortunately, these types of facilities exist only in the private sector.

How to begin a sustainable lifestyle with mental illness? You begin by coping with your fears. Secondly, not allowing life's uncertainties to take control of your thought process. Third, initiating a strong belief system and surrounding yourself with positive people as well as joining a support group. It is imperative that you make the necessary and recommended lifestyle changes such as dissolving disruptive relationships. Changing your current environment or those who help play a role in inducing or producing a negative impact on your life.

Remember, the initiation of a new relation or environment can have just as much a negative impact on your coping ability as your old ones. Your individual actions, as well as your reactions to the stimulus, play an essential role. Response and response time to the stimulus also will play a major role in your quick recovery from a crisis. Therefore, continue to identify and eliminate each stressor that serves as a source for mood destabilization.

However, there will be times when those unforeseen events will show up and disrupt your life. You absolutely cannot allow these events to usher you into a crisis. Learn how to properly react or respond appropriately to such triggers. Do not allow this one event or sequence of events to have a major or negative impact on your life. Immediately get in touch with your support team, family members, or spiritual advisor for help.

Time and time again, I have overheard psychologist tells their patients to avoid the negative self-talk. Learn to stand in the mirror and remind yourself just how wondrous God has created you. Point out all the wonderful qualities that you love about yourself such as physical attributes, facial characteristics, height, or length of hair. Do all those wonderful things that will help you feel attractive, warm (beautiful or handsome). Remember you are doing all these wonderful things for yourself and not to achieve the approval of others.

Another wonderful practice is to constantly remind yourself of all the small and great things that you have accomplished in your life. Whether it is a successful marriage, raising children, starting a business, or obtaining a degree or a new skill. Remember to reward yourself often for such accomplishments. In addition to this, join a new club, social organization, or church group. Attend therapeutic sessions that will aid you in achieving your best. One that will aid you in becoming whole again.

Avoid alcohol consumption, when possible, because alcohol consumption and mood stabilizers do not match. All too often, there is that individual who will restart or turn back to old habits thinking that they are stable enough to an adapt with drugs and alcohol. On the contrary, alcohol and drug consumption along with mood stabilizers will often trigger an adverse reaction. Many of these adverse reactions can turn out to be fatal. So do not mix drugs or alcohol with your medication regime.

Chapter Twenty-Five
Overcoming Strength

Recently, I read an article that quoted several of the comments made by their participants. However, there was one comment made by a participant that really struck a chord. The individual stated the following, "only whites have the luxury to sit around and talk. Blacks have to keep moving to stay alive." I would like to deem this statement as factional. Most working-class African Americans cannot afford the luxury of withdrawing from steady employment to pursue six or seven months of mental health recovery. Absence from work can sometimes result in a loss of wages. Moreover, it could result in permanent dismissal.

Today, very few employers will offer insurance coverage. Let alone offer a policy that provides compensation for lengthy outpatient therapy. Once the employer gains knowledge of the nature of the illness, nine times out of ten the employee will be dismissed from the job. Ms. Lillie was one of those individuals who has repeatedly received job dismissal due to her recurring mental illness. However, she did not allow this to prevent her from regaining her momentum.

Once released from the hospital, she would jump right back on the bandwagon and return to work. No matter what Ms. Lillie endured, she continued to bounce back into the workforce. There was nothing that society could throw at Ms. Lillie that would keep her from achieving her goals.

Chapter Twenty-Six

Stigma

Let us now discuss one of the greatest assaults and contributors of the past. This contributor/assault came in the form of stigma. One that single-handedly prevented many African Americans from receiving proper mental health treatment. The contributor that I am referring to is a cultural stigma. Cultural stigma was the assailant that caused millions of Americans to forfeit proper mental health treatment. What exactly is stigma? A stigma is defined as "a mark of disgrace associated with circumstance, quality or person." I shared this bit of knowledge with you to demonstrate how culture can really have a greater impact on someone's mental health status (Matthew, Corrigan, Smith, Aranda, 2006).

Unfortunately, the stigma as an assailant did not stand alone. The stigmas were directly associated with ignorance—the lack of knowledge concerning mental illness and information regarding establishing a proper treatment. There were several of us who lived within the same community, who walked in constant shame of this because one or both of our parents suffered from mental illness.

When you are growing up in a predominately African American community, there are many cultural norms as well as abnormal behaviors that are accepted. For instance, blasting your music or observing a couple fighting on the sidewalk. These are classified as so-called normal behaviors. However, there is one abnormal behavior that is now widely accepted, yet when I was growing up it was considered as an omen. This widely unaccepted behavior was called manic depression.

Whenever someone in my neighborhood displayed abnormal behavior, they were deemed a drug addict or simply crazy. Ms. Lillie was deemed "crazy." Oftentimes, the neighborhood children would not only mock me, but they would also mock my mother. We could hardly walk down the street without overhearing harsh comments being whispered among our neighbors.

Other times, the neighborhood children would walk behind Ms. Lillie mimicking her every gesture. Including the way she walked and talked. My mother had spent many years in Los Angeles and therefore acquired a very distinctive dialect.

A Final Note

Despite modern intervention, millions of Americans suffer in silence with mental illness because of the stigma surrounding those who are affected by this illness. One-third of these individuals will seek out and receive excellent care through the private sector. While another one-third will sit by and suffer in silence or receive poor to little mental health care. This book was written in hopes to help the people who have endured this dreadful illness and the horrific effects which it exerts on the family.

Nevertheless the issue remains that there are not enough public institutions who provide such fantastic and award-winning services to moderate to low-income individuals who suffer or struggle with mental illness. However, living with mental illness is not a solution; it is an addendum to the problem. Now is the time to come up with a solution to the problem. And that problem is how do I live with mental illness.

References

Youngman-Coleman, Sydney RN, BSN, RNC

Mayo Foundation for Medical Education and Research, "Healthy Lifestyle Stress management" 1998-2016 ed.

Lancer Darlene JD, MFT (Licensed Marriage and Family Therapist)

What Are Personal Boundaries? How Do I Get Some? http://psychcentral.com/lib/what-are-personal-boundaries-how-do-i-get-some.

Matthews, Alicia K, Corrigan Patrick W., Smith A, Barbara M, Aranda, Frances. A Qualitative Exploration of African-Americans' Attitude Toward Mental Illness and Mental Illness Treatment Seeking

Manderscheid Ronald W., Ph.D., Director, Ryff Carol D., Ph.D., Elsie J. Freeman, MD, MPH, McKnight-Eily Lela R., Ph.D., Dhingra Satvinder, MPH, Strine Tara W., MPH. Evolving Definitions of Mental Illness and Wellness: Prev Chronic Dis. 2010 Jan; 7(1): A19.Published online 2009 December 15.

Judd LL, Akiskal HS, Zeller PJ, Paulus M, Leon AC, Maser JD, et al. Psychosocial disability during the long-term course of unipolar major depressive disorder. Arch Gen Psychiatry. 2000;57(4):375–380. [PubMed]

Goodwin FK, Jamison KR. Bipolar disorder and recurrent depression, 2nd edition. New York (NY): Oxford University Press; 2007.

Diagnostic and, statistical, 4th edition, text revision. Diagnostic and statistical manual of mental disorders.4th edition, text revision. Washington (DC): American Psychiatric Association; 2000.

Keller MB, Shapiro RW, Lavori PW, Wolfe N. Relapse in major depressive disorder: analysis with the life table. Arch Gen Psychiatry. 1982;39(8):911–915. [PubMed]

Aspinwall LG, Staudinger UM. A psychology of human strengths: perspectives on an emerging field. Washington (DC): American Psychiatric Association; 2002.

Primm AB, Vasquez MJT, Mays RA, Sammons-Posey D, McKnight-Eily LR, Presley-Cantrell LR, et al. The role of public health in addressing racial and ethnic disparities in mental health and mental illness. Dis. 2010 7(1) http://www.cdc.gov/pcd/issues/2010/jan/09_0125. htm. [PMC free article] [PubMed]